ANTI INFL

MW00880323

DIET

BEGINNER'S GUIDE: WHAT YOU NEED TO KNOW TO HEAL YOURSELF WITH FOOD, RESTORE OVERALL HEALTH AND BECOME PAIN FREE + RECIPES + 7 DAYS DIET PLAN

INTRODUCTION

I want to thank you and congratulate you for getting the book, *"Anti-Inflammatory Diet"*.

Inflammation. When we hear this word, we always associate it with the swelling of the muscles, usually in our joints. Our usual remedies for this is to take a pain reliever, apply anti-inflammation ointments and oils and or apply hot or cold compress. These remedies are only for ordinary inflammation, which result from our body's instinct to prevent infection.

However, there are inflammation diseases that are chronic, which means that tissues in our body swells even if they are not preventing any infection. Most of these chronic inflammations happen in our internal organs, which we do not get to notice. Thus, putting us in greater danger. Chronic inflammation is the cause of some of the most common fatal diseases among adults.

For chronic inflammation diseases, one of the best remedies is to change your diet. Food can trigger or increase the risk of inflammations in our organ. Knowing what to eat and what to avoid may help you lower the risk and may manage your chronic inflammations. Preventing food related inflammation will have long-term health benefits to those who engage in this diet regimen.

This book contains information about chronic inflammation and how to avoid or reduce the risk of having it and how to manage it, if you are diagnosed to have diseases that causes inflammations. It provide the food that you need to eat, may eat and should not eat. As a bonus, it will provide you with the list of the food, which helps prevent inflammations. In addition, there is also a 7-day meal plan to help you start with your diet and some healthy and hearty recipes that you may include in your meal planning.

Thanks again for getting this book. I hope you enjoy it!

TABLE OF CONTENTS

CHAPTER 1

THE PRINCIPLES OF ANTI-INFLAMMATORY DIET

Inflammation is the body's natural reaction towards infection or injury. When observed from the outside, inflammation can be described by its signs and symptoms like redness, heat coming out of the tissue, pain and increase in the size of the tissue. We are all too familiar with this signs and symptoms. We see them in people with allergies or who have been injured.

When bacteria enter the body for example, and damage some of our cells, the cells release certain chemicals that signal to the body that there is a problem. The chemicals released cause the signs and symptoms that we are familiar with. The combined effects of the chemicals histamine and bradykinin for example, cause pain. Histamine, together with prostaglandin, is also responsible for the accumulation of fluid in the area, which causes swelling. The actions of these chemicals are meant to limit the damage caused by the foreign body that has entered our system.

The presence of the inflammation chemicals in the bloodstream also creates some changes in the walls of the blood vessels. This allows certain types of white blood cells to enter the inflamed tissue to destroy the microorganism causing the damage.

The white blood cells play a vital role in the inflammatory response. The first time your immune system encounter a certain foreign body, it tries to destroy it and create special types of cells, called Plasma cells. This type of white blood cell has one purpose -- to identify the new threat if ever more of it enters the body again.

The plasma cells create antibodies. These proteins found in the blood are designed to attach to the surface of the foreign body. Their attachment to the foreign body triggers an immune response towards the said foreign body. One of the common immune responses is inflammation.

WHEN THINGS DO NOT GO AS EXPECTED

There are times when this defense mechanism works against us. In the case of people with rheumatoid arthritis for example, we see the signs of inflammation in their joints. There is no foreign organism or particles in these joints. The immune system in this case, is attacking the body's own functional tissues. Somewhere along the way, it made a mistake and created antibodies against the body's own tissues. When this happens, health professionals call the condition an autoimmune disorder.

There are also times when the state of inflammation goes on even when there is no more threat in the body. Some of the chemicals that are supposed to signal the stop of inflammation are never released into the blood stream. There are some instances when some types of proteins that promote inflammation stay in the blood stream too long. This keeps the body in constant alert, maintaining the state of inflammation even when it is not needed.

CHRONIC INFLAMMATION AND ITS ROLE IN CREATING DISEASES

There are two types of inflammation, acute and chronic. They differ in the length of time that they are activated. When we eat something that we are allergic to, we show signs of inflammation for a few hours or even days. As soon as the allergen is out of our system, we go back to normal. This is an example of acute inflammation.

Some types of inflammation last for longer periods. When we have an infection that is not cured for example, the inflammation in the infected area may remain for weeks or months. This is an example of chronic inflammation. Some types of chronic inflammation do not even create pain, making the person think that everything is okay. He is not aware that the immune system is working in the background even when there is no immediate threat to his health.

Because inflammation also spends a lot of energy, it may cause a person to feel fatigue. Long-term chronic inflammation can cause the body to be in a constant state of stress. An inflammation in one part of the body may create more in other parts. Most of the time, we do not feel them happening because we do not see the usual signs of illness. However, over a long period of chronic inflammation, diseases that are more serious may form. Undetected chronic inflammation for example, has been linked to various heart diseases. More studies are being conducted to establish links to other common fatal diseases that we associate with age, such as stroke and vascular diseases.

CHAPTER 2

DISEASES AND HEALTH CONDITIONS RELATED TO INFLAMMATION

Doctors are now discovering that inflammation plays major roles in the development of many common chronic diseases.

Chronic diseases are non-contagious illnesses that last for years. Unlike infections, one particular foreign body does not cause them. This makes them more difficult to cure. Some examples of chronic diseases are diabetes, cardiovascular diseases, arthritis and cancer. When they happen, they are there for the long term. When they are present, it is difficult to completely undo them. When it comes to chronic diseases, prevention is the best remedy.

Most people never get the chance to learn about these chronic diseases. They spend their days not thinking about the types and quantities of food they eat and their level of activity. Some even increase their chances of getting these chronic diseases by doing vices that they know are bad of their health.

Because of this, chronic diseases in general accounts for more than 70 percent of the deaths in developed countries. More than 130 million Americans have one type of chronic disease. 60% of these people have more than one chronic disease. These numbers are from the Centers of Disease Control. Their data come only from reported cases. The number is growing every day.

If you examine every type of chronic disease, you will find that all of them have some form of inflammation. Rheumatoid arthritis for example is the inflammation of the joints. Pancreatitis is the inflammation of the pancreas because the immune system is attacking the pancreatic cells.

HEART ATTACKS AND

INFLAMMATION

Heart diseases happen because of atherosclerosis or the accumulation of plaques in the inner walls of the blood vessels. This rarely happens without being worsened by chronic inflammation.

In systemic inflammation, there are multiple points of inflammation is blood vessels all over our bodies. When a part of the blood vessels become damaged and inflamed, the body repairs it by covering it with a layer of cholesterol. This is what we refer to as plaque. With chronic inflammation, the blood vessels are always inflamed. Because of this, the body keeps placing layers of cholesterol to patch up the inflamed surfaces. This leads to the narrowing of the blood vessels. When the blood vessels become narrow, they are more prone to blockage of solid particles like clotted blood.

DIABETES AND INFLAMMATION

Diabetes is characterized by high glucose levels. For most people, the high glucose levels happen because of insulin resistance of various cells and tissues in the body.

The level of our blood sugar has an effect on our immune system. When the blood sugar level is elevated, the release of certain chemicals is triggered. These chemicals weaken your immune system and it initiates systemic inflammation. When tissues are in an inflamed state, they are less receptive to insulin. This prevents the glucose from entering the body, further increasing the blood sugar level. The chain reaction continues to increase the blood sugar level and the intensity of inflammation.

CANCERS AND INFLAMMATION

Cancer cells are a mutation of regular cells. A part of these cells' DNA has changed and this causes it to multiply itself. Chronic inflammation causes DNA changes in cells. Some of these DNA changes may lead to cancer.

Recurring inflammations caused by infections can also alter the arrangement of DNA. This may also lead to certain types of cancer. Cervical cancer for example is caused by the Human Papillomavirus. Hepatitis-causing viruses can also cause liver cancer.

CHRONIC KIDNEY DISEASES AND INFLAMMATION

The body can suffer from inflammation due to chronic kidney disease. People suffering from uremia and undergoing hemodialysis are at a high risk of getting inflammation in their muscles because the body breaks it down to supply more protein in some parts of the body.

Due to uremia, the creatinine level increases and may cause chronic inflammation, which may eventually lead to heart disease. Along with the increase of the creatinine level, the albumin level decreases. The low level of albumin may cause inflammation in the legs or arms.

These are only some of the common forms of chronic diseases that are related to inflammation. Inflammation also plays a role in the development of many other chronic diseases. This is the reason that we need to take measures to decrease the chances of inflammation occurring in our body.

CHAPTER 3

FOOD AND INFLAMMATION

Most people are not aware that the things that they take into their bodies start certain degrees of inflammation. When a person smokes for example, the presence of tar in his lungs create a perpetual state of inflammation there.

The same happens when we eat certain foods that our body rejects. Some people for example, do not have the capacity to digest foods with lactose. This happens because their body does not produce the specific enzyme used to digest this form of carbohydrate. Because of the body sees lactose as a foreign substance that does not belong to the digestive tract, it initiates the inflammation process. The person feels pain, which is one of the cardinal signs of inflammation. Though we cannot see what it happening, we can only imagine the other signs of inflammation in his digestive tract.

THE DIGESTIVE ORGANS AS A PRIORITY FOR THE IMMUNE SYSTEM

The immune system is the security force of our body, and one of its most important protective assignments is the gastro-intestinal tract. This is the tract where our food passes as it is digested. Along the tracts, there is a system of tissues designed to monitor and act on threats that may enter the body. In the medical field, this is referred to as the Gut Associated Lymphoid Tissue or GALT. The GALT comprises more than 70% of our whole immune system.

When there is a foreign substance in our digestive tract, the components of the immune system in the GALT become active an initiate the immune response. Because of this, we need to watch what we eat. We need to make sure that the food that we put in out body will not make our immune system react.

CREATING A DIET PLAN THAT IS IN HARMONY WITH YOUR IMMUNE SYSTEM

Our goal is to create a diet plan that does not initiate the inflammatory process from the immune system. Unlike most diet plans, the goal with this one is not weight loss. With this plan, there is no end goal. It is a lifetime diet plan because the need to fight systemic inflammation increases as we become older.

We should start organizing your anti-inflammatory diet by listing down the types of food that you should not eat. These types of foods induce inflammation.

Food that have high level of Sugar

As stated in the previous chapter, high blood sugar levels put certain cells in the inflammatory state. Because of this, you should limit the amount of sugar that you take in. When looking for sweeteners, you should look for natural substitutes to processed sugar. Examples of substitute sweeteners are pure maple syrup and agave nectar.

Food rich in carbohydrates

Aside from sucrose (sugar) you should also other forms of carbohydrates that you consume in a regular basis. All types of bread for example are full of starch. Consuming an excess of starch regularly will increase your stored carbs and your blood sugar. It also does not give your body an opportunity to burn off excess fats and other forms of stored energy.

Food high in Trans Fats

Trans fats are found in many fried foods. They can be found in common fried foods in fast food restaurants. Trans fats contribute to inflammation because they lowers the levels of good cholesterol and increase the levels of bad cholesterol in the blood stream. They also increase the chance of obesity and insulin resistance.

Food that are rich in Omega-6

Omega 6 is a type of fatty acid that is found in vegetable and canola oils. Diets that are high in this fatty acid are highly inflammatory for most people. These types of diets have also been associated with common cancers.

You should also keep track of the foods that you are sensitive to. Here are some food substances that a lot of people are allergic to:

- Milk and other dairy products
- Seafood

- Gluten

- Chicken

- Nuts

If you are allergic to these, you should avoid them at all costs to prevent onset of inflammation inside your body.

When designing your own meal plan, you should stick to organic products. Try to satisfy your hunger with whole foods and green leafy vegetables rather than carbohydrate-rich foods. You should also choose foods with a lot of omega-3. Right now, the best food source for this nutrient is deep ocean fishes like tuna. If you don't have access to foods with this nutrient, you can also take fish oil supplements. You should also have your blood chemistry checked regularly. One of the common causes of inflammation is the imbalance in substances found in the blood. You should then adjust your diet according to your results.

Food that increases the cholesterol level

Cholesterol in the blood level increases the risk of having a heart attack. When the blood is high in cholesterol, the LDL or low-density lipoprotein is absorbed by the artery. To stop the absorption, the arteries swells. This result to an increase accumulation of cholesterol in the arteries, which can cause or worsen cardiovascular diseases.

Food that are high in purine

Purine breaks into uric acid when processed by the body. The muscles need uric acid to function and develop well. However, high level of uric acid in the blood can cause inflammation. The inflammation results to gout and arthritis in the joints.

Now that you know about what food to avoid, you can now develop a list of food that may help you plan your diet. Below is a sample list of the foods you are allowed to eat, you are limited to eat and you should avoid.

FOODS YOU ARE ALLOWED TO EAT A

LOT

- All non-highly processed rice and cereals

- Brocolli, artichokes, cabbage and endives

- Carrots, cucumber, eggplant

- Pumpking, squash and zucchini

- Beets, sweet potatoes, white (regular) potatoes*

- Turnips

- All plain breads

- Skim milk

- All kinds of fresh fruits

- All fresh herbs and spices

- Egg whites

- Vegetable stocks

- All unsweetened or fresh fruit juice and fruit sorbets which are not made from citrus fruits

- Teas

*Double boil these root crops to lessen the potassium. Too much potassium may help increase creatinine in your blood. High level of creatinine may cause inflammation in your kidneys and result to uremia.

FOODS YOU SHOULD EAT IN MODERATION (4X A WEEK)

- Chicken without the skin

- Seafoods

- Tuna, bluefish, herring, salmon and white fishes

- Crab, lobster and oysters

- Asparagus, and cauliflower

- Corn and corn products

- Spinach, kale and other dark green vegetables (Studies show that dark green vegetables have moderate purine content.)

- Any kinds of mushroom

- Tomatoes

- Chicken stocks

- Coffee (regular, americano and latte*)

- Cocoa and low fat milk drinks

- Healthy oils, e.g. olive oil, coconut oil, sesame oil

- Citrus fruit juices

*Milk used should be low-fat or skim milk.

FOODS THAT YOU SHOULD EAT

LIGHTLY (2X A WEEK)

- Venison, rabbit, lamb, pork and other red meat. Consumption should not exceed 4 ounces a day.

- Whole eggs

- Butter and margarine, palm oil, corn oil, canola oil

- Egg noodles and pasta made from whole wheat

- Squab, duck, turkey, pigeon and pheasant. These birds are high in protein, but are rich in cholesterol and purine.

- Halibut and trout. These fishes are high in purine.

- Shrimps, mussels and other shellfishes

- Chicken liver

- Meat stocks

- Lentils and bean products *No*

- Cheeses and yogurts. Consumption should be limited to 100 grams a day. *No*

- Carbonated drinks except for colas. Consumption should be limited to 8 ounces a day *No*

- Beers and wine

- Special coffee e.g. espresso, mojito, capuccino.

FOOD YOU SHOULD AVOID

COMPLETELY

- Anchovies and sardines. These are high in purine

- Pork and pork stocks. These are high in fats and cholesterol.

- Processed foods

- Shortenings, lards and animal oils

- Meat liver

- Chicken skin

- Brain, kidneys and lungs of livestocks

- Gravies and condiments

- Colas

- Whole milk

After a month of focusing on these types of food, you will feel stronger and some of your chronic inflammations may subside.

CHAPTER 4

7-DAY ANTI-INFLAMMATION MEAL PLAN

With the help of the previous chapter, here is a 7-day anti-inflammation meal which you may follow.vThis 7-day anti-inflammation meal plan may make use of some of the recipes suggested in the next chapter. If you find that some of the berries, fruits, vegetables or other ingredients are not available in your area, you can easily replace them with the ones that are in season or their appropriate substitutes.

DAY 1

Breakfast

1 serving of Banana Cashew Toast

1 cup of coffee or tomato juice

Total Calories: 380

Lunch

Chicken and vegetable salad

1 pita bread

1 cup of fresh fruit juice

Total Calories: 540

Dinner

Broiled White fish

Zucchini spaghetti with Pesto sauce

1 cup of fresh fruit juice or wine

Total calories 580

Snacks

1 cup berries

Total calories: 120

DAY 2

Breakfast

1 serving of white egg fritata with brocolli

1 cup of tea, or fresh fruit juice

Total calories: 240

Lunch

1 serving of cucumber-mango salad

Grilled cod

Total calories: 490

Dinner

Broiled chicken served with rice

Vegetable soup

1 cup of fresh juice

Total calories: 510

Snacks

2 Hearty Blueberry muffin

Total calories: 300

DAY 3

Breakfast

Apple Cinnamon oatmeal

1 cup of coffee or tea

Total Calories: 280

Lunch

Chicken curry served with rice

1 banana

1 cup fresh juice

Total Calories:570

Dinner

Baked fillet mignon with potato

½ cup grapes

1 cup fruit juice*

Total calories: 620

Snacks

½ cup of cashew, walnut or almonds

Total calories: 400

DAY 4

Breakfast

1 serving sweet potato hash with eggs

1 cup of skim milk, tea or coffee

Total Calories: 310

Lunch

Baked marinated tofu served Spiced lemon salad

1 cup fresh juice

Total calories: 465

Dinner

Steamed Grilled Salmon with Cilantro sauce

1 cup cauliflower rice

1/8 wedge of small cantaloupe

Total calories: 610

Snacks

1 200 grams of carrot or celery sticks with avocado dip

Total Calories: 280

DAY 5

Breakfast

Swiss Chard and Spinach with Egg

1 toasted pita bread

1 cup of milk, coffee or tea

Total calories: 310

Lunch

1 serving Chicken noodle soup

1 banana or grapefruit

Total calories: 330

Dinner

Baked Chicken and Fruits

1 cup rice

1 cup fresh fruit juice

Total calories: 630

Snacks

1 large apple

Total Calories: 110

DAY 6

Breakfast

2 serving of French Toast serve with slices of banana

1 cup of non-fat or milk, tea or coffee

Total calories: 350

Lunch

Seasoned Salmon in Olive oil with rice

1 cup of fresh fruit juice

Total calories: 410

Dinner

Greek Couscous

Grouper fillet with Tamarind Base Fish Consomme

1 cup of green tea

Total calories: 560

Snacks

Boiled squash and okra

Total calories: 80

DAY 7

Breakfast

Blended Coconut Milk and Banana Breakfast smoothie

Lunch

Baked Chicken with vegetables and seasoning

½ cup rice

1 cup of fresh fruit juice

Dinner

Baked Tilapia with rice

1 cup white wine or iced tea or any fruit juice

Snacks

Oven Crisp Sweet potatoes

Total Calories: 90

You can also interchange some meals. You can reserve the hot meals on cold nights for example. There is no need to follow this meal to the letter. This meal plan is meant to be used merely as a guide when you choose your own dishes to prepare. The following chapter will provide you some recipes to get you started.

CHAPTER 5

ANTI-INFLAMMATION MEAL RECIPES

This chapter gives you the recipes included in the 7-day meal plan.

BREAKFAST

Banana Cashew Toast

Serves 4 with 330 calories per serving

Ingredients:

- 1 cup roasted cashews (unsalted)
- 4 pieces oat bread
- 2 ripe medium-sized bananas
- Dash of salt

- Pinch of cinnamon

- 2 tsp. flax meals

- 2 tsp. honey

Instructions:

Peel and slice the bananas into ½-inch pieces. Toast the bread. In a food processor, puree the salt and cashews until they are smooth. Use the puree as a spread on the toasts. On top of the spread, arrange a layer of bananas. Add flax meals and a dash of cinnamon on top of the bananas. Top the toast with honey.

Blended Coconut Milk and Banana Breakfast Smoothie

Serves 4 adults with 330 calories per serving

Ingredients:

- 4 ripe medium sized bananas
- 4 tbsp. flax seeds
- 2 cups almond milk
- 2 cups coconut milk
- 4 tsp. cinnamon

Instructions:

Peel the banana and slice it into ½-inch pieces. Put all the ingredients in the blender and blend into a smoothie. Add a dash of cinnamon at the top of the smoothie before serving.

Strawberry Yogurt treat

Serves 4 with 310 calories per serving

Ingredients:

- 4 cups 0% fat plain yogurt

- 1 cup sliced strawberries

- 8 tbsp. of flax meal

- 4 tbsp. honey

- 8 tbsp. walnuts (chopped)

Instructions:

Distribute 2 cups of the yogurt into your serving bowls. Neatly layer the flax meal and the walnut in the middle. Add a drizzle of half of the honey before covering with the last layer of yogurt. Add the honey on top of the yogurt to add color when you serve.

Omega-3-rich Cold Banana Breakfast

Serves 2 adults with 350 calories per serving

Ingredients:

- ½ cup cold milk

- 4 tbsp. sesame seeds

- 2 tbsp. flaxseeds

- 4 tbsp. sunflower seeds

- 2 tbsp. ground coconut

- 1 sliced large Banana

Instructions:

Mix the milk and honey on your breakfast bowl. Use your coffee grinder to grind all the seeds. Add the ground seeds to the honey and milk mixture. Place the sliced bananas neatly on top. Sprinkle the ground coconuts for added flavor.

Swiss Chard and Spinach with Egg

Serves 4 with 160 calories per serving

Ingredients:

- 4 egg whites

- 4 pieces of rice bread

- 20 pieces spinach leaves

- 20 pieces Swiss chard leaves

- 4 tbsp. parsley (fresh)

- 1 tsp. olive oil

- Sea salt, ground pepper and dried mint

Instructions:

Heat 2 cups of water in a pan just below the boiling point. Open an egg, separate the whites from the yolks. Put the whites in small bowl. Lower the bowl towards the heated water and gently pour the egg into the pan. Do the same with the other eggs. Poach the eggs for 4 minutes. After that, gently take the eggs, one at a time and transfer them into a plate. Do the same with the remaining 2 eggs.

Chop the parsley and sauté the leaves in a pan for 6 minutes. Toast the bread while doing this. When done, make a layer of the sautéed greens and the chopped parsley on top of the toasted rice bread. Place the poached eggs on top of the bed of greens. Sprinkle each serving with ground pepper, sea salt and dried mint.

Egg white Fritata with Brocolli

Serves 1 with 140 calories

Ingredients:

- 4 egg whites
- 1 teaspoon olive oil
- 1 small clove of garlic, minced
- ½ of medium sized shallot, minced
- ½ teaspon fresh thyme, chopped
- ½ cup brocolli, chopped into tiny flowerettes or strips
- ¼ teaspoon of salt
- pepper

Instructions:

In a bowl, whisk together the egg whites, salt and thyme.

Place a non-stick skillet over medium heat. Pour the olive oil.

Saute the onion until it becomes translucent in color. Add the garlic and saute for another two or five minutes.

Stir in the brocolli until tender. This will take about 3 to 5 minutes. Lower the heat.

Pour the egg white mixture over the brocolli and let it set for about 2 minutes. Flip the fritata and cook for another minute.

Season with pepper and additional salt to taste.

Apple Oatmeal

Serves 2 with 220 calories per serving

Ingredients:

- 2/3 cups rolled oats

- 1 cup water

- 1 teaspoon ground cinnamon

- 1 cup of any non-fat milk, coconut milk or almond milk (optional)

- ¼ cup fresh apple juice

- 1 chopped apple, (unpeeled or peeled)

Instructions

Place the water, juice and the apple in a deep pot. Bring to boil over medium heat.

Add the oats and cinnamon. Bring to another boil. Lower the heat and let it simmer for 3 minutes or until it is thick.

Divide the serving into two and serve with milk.

Sweet Potato Hash

Serves 2 with 240 calories per serving

Ingredients:

- 2 cupes sweet potatoes, cut in bite size pieces

- 1 small sized red onion, minced

- 2 garlic cloves, minced

- ¼ cup chopped chives

- 1 bell pepper, diced

- 1 tablespoon coconut oil

- Salt and pepper

- 4 egg whites, (optional)

Instructions:

Heat the oil in a skillet, placed over medium heat. Saute the onion until translucent. Add the garlic and saute for another minute. Stir in the sweet potatoes and cook for 10 minutes.

Put in the bell pepper and chives. Reserve a teapoon of chives for garnishing.

Cook for another 5 minutes or until the sweet potato turns soft and golden brown. Divide the potatoes into two servings.

Whisk the egg whites with salt and pepper. Place a different skillet over medium heat. Add 1 teaspoon of olive oil and lower the heat. Pour the egg whites evenly on the skillet. Let it settle for two minutes. Turn off the fire and cover the skillet for twenty seconds.

Turn the egg whites over a wide plate and roll it from one end to another. Divide the egg in a half. Cut the egg whites in ½ inch strip and place on top of the hash.

Garnish with the chives. Serve.

*Note: You can substitute cubed tofu for the eggs.

French Toast

Serves 4 with 127 calories per serving

Ingredients:

- 1 egg white

- 4 thick slices of white bread

- 1 teaspoon sugar

- 1/3 cup almond milk or skim milk

- Dash of cinnamon

- Dash of salt

- 1 tablespoon all-purpose flour

- ¼ teaspoon of vanilla extract

- 1 tablespoon of coconut oil

Instructions:

Place the flour in a bowl. Gradually, add the milk until the flour is dissolved. Stir in the egg, cinnamon, salt, vanilla and sugar. Mix thoroughly.

Heat a griddle pan over medium heat. Grease the pan with coconut oil.

Soak the bread slices in the egg mixture until the mixture is absorbed. Arrange the bread slices in the griddle pan. Cook the bread slices until they are golden brown or about 3 minutes on each side.

Serve with slices of banana or strawberry. Or drizzle maple syrup over it.

LUNCH

Spiced Lemon Salad

Serves 2 adults with 150 calories per serving

Ingredients:

- 2 cups of shredded lettuce

- 4 medium sized lemons

- ¼ cup honey

- ½ tsp. sea salt

- A pinch of Cayenne pepper

Instructions:

Place your lettuce in your salad bowl. Extract the juice from 3 and a half of the lemons. For the last half, grate it to get around 1 teaspoon of grated lemon zest. In another bowl, mix the juice, the honey, the salt and pepper. Pour it over the prepared lettuce shreds and toss. Top it with the shredded lemon zest.

Spinach and Avocado Salad

Serves 5 with 470 calories per serving

Ingredients:

Salad dressing:

- 1 cup extra virgin olive oil

- ½ cup honey

- ½ tsp. Dijon mustard

- ½ cup red wine vinegar

- ½ tsp. paprika

- 1 ½ tsp. dried onions

- 3 tbsp. sesame seeds

- 1 ½ tbsp. poppy seeds

  Salad:

- 300 grams of spinach leaves (fresh)

- 2-3 pieces avocados (medium sized)

- 1 cup toasted almonds (straight cut)

Instructions:

In a mixing bowl, mix all the liquid ingredients of the dressing. Mince the dried onions and ground the seeds using a coffee grinder. Leave a pinch of seeds for toppings. Add the remaining solid ingredients of the dressing in the mixing bowl and mix.

Wash and chop the spinach and drain the water. Remove the seeds from the avocados and scrape the meat off the fruit. Cut the avocado meat into bitesize pieces. Place the spinach and the avocados in your salad bowl. Pour the dressing mixture over it and toss.

Sprinkle the almonds and the remaining seeds on the top of the tossed salad.

Anti-inflammation Chicken Curry

Serves 4 with 370 calories per serving

Ingredients:

- 1 onion (medium)

- 3 cloves garlic

- ¾ tbsp. extra-virgin olive oil

- 4-5 carrots

- 330 grams organic chicken broth

- 550 grams of organic chicken breasts (skinless and boneless)

- 300 grams coconut milk

- 3 tsp. Curry powder

- 1 ½ tsp. Ginger powder

Instructions:

Chop the onion, slice the carrots into sticks and mince the garlic cloves. In a medium heat, you should then sauté the half of the olive oil, onion and garlic. After a couple of minutes, add the carrots.

You should then sauté the chicken in a separate skillet using what remains of the oil. When the carrots are cooked, add the coconut milk and broth. When the liquid has settled, add the sautéed chicken.

Add the powders to taste. Let the flavor of the powders penetrate the meat as the chicken cooks. This takes around 7-9 minutes. Serve hot.

Baked marinated tofu

Serves 2 with 275 calories per serving

Ingredients:

- 300 grams tofu (extra firm)

- 1 ½ tbsp. sesame oil

- 1 ½ tbsp. tamari (wheat-free)

- 1 ½ tbsp. unprocessed honey

- 1 garlic clove

- 1 tsp. fresh ginger (grated)

Instructions:

You should do this first set of instructions a full day before the meal. Drain the tofu adequately. When thoroughly dried, slice the tofu into slabs. In a bowl, mix the tamari, garlic, honey, ginger and the oil. Place the sliced tofu in the bowl with the mixture. Make sure that the tofu slices are all submerged in the marinade. Seal the top of the bowl with a plastic wrap.

On the day of the meal, place the tofu slices on a baking sheet then bake at 374°F. Let it bake for 12 minutes. Turn the tofu to bake the other side for the same length of time.

Seasoned Salmon in Olive oil

Serves 4 with 200 calories per serving

Ingredients:

- 350 grams wild salmon (Filleted)
- 1 tbsp. extra-virgin olive oil

Seasoning

- 2 tsp. sea salt
- 1/2 tsp. ground black pepper
- 1 ½ tbsp. garlic powder
- 3 tsp. cayenne pepper
- 3 tbsp. mixed dried parsley flakes and dried basil
- 3 tsp. thyme

Instructions:

In a mixing bowl, combine all the seasoning ingredients and mix. Make a layer of the seasoning mixture on a plate. Let each side of the salmon touch the layer of seasoning. Make sure that there is even coating in each side of the salmon.

Using low-medium heat, you should pre-heat the olive oil in a pan. Place the fish right before the oil starts to show fumes. Let it cook and turn it after 3 ½ minutes. Continue cooking and flipping until the fish is cooked to your preference.

This is best served with vinegar dressing.

Chicken soup in almonds and coconuts

Serves 4 with 500 calories per serving

Ingredients:

- 3 pieces green onions

- 3 cloves of garlic

- 1 ½ tsp. extra virgin olive oil

- ¼ cup smooth almond butter

- 2/3 cup light coconut milk

- 1 ½ tbsp. fresh lemon juice

- 1 ½ tbsp. wheat-free tamari

- 2/3 tbsp. fish sauce

- 1/4 cup water

- 550 grams organic chicken breasts (Skinless)

- 1 large head of broccoli with stalk

- 150 grams rice noodles (the thinnest you can find)

- ½ cup roasted nuts

- ½ cup dried cranberries

Instructions:

Chop the onions to separate the white parts. Those are the only ones that we will need. Mince the garlic and chop the chicken into cubes. Also, chop the broccoli into smaller pieces.

Cook the noodles according to the package directions. In a saucepan, you should sauté the garlic and onion using extra virgin olive oil. Put the coconut milk, lemon juice, almond butter, tamari, fish sauce and water in a blender and blend. When the mixture is smooth add the cooked garlic and onion and keep continue to blend.

Put the blended mixture in a heated large pan. Add in the chicken then the broccoli. Cover in medium heat for about 12-15 minutes. Add the cooked noodles, berries and the nuts right before you serve.

Baked Chicken with vegetables and seasoning

Serves 4 with 520 calories per serving

Ingredients:

- ½ cup rice wine vinegar

- 1 cup chicken broth

- 1 tbsp. miso paste

- ½ tsp. dried thyme

- ½ tbsp. garlic powder

- 1 medium onion, sliced

- 300 grams of yams, sliced

- 4 medium carrots, quartered,

- 6 pieces organic chicken breasts (boneless and skinless)

- 2 tbsp. extra virgin olive oil

- 1 1/2 tbsp. dried parsley

- ½ tsp of cayenne pepper

Instructions:

Slice the onion, yams and carrots. Arrange them in a baking dish. Preheat the oven at 246 C. Mix the vinegar, broth, miso paste, dried thyme, and the garlic powder. Organize the chicken on top of the arranged vegetables in the baking dish. On top of the chicken, pour the broth mixture. Add the olive oil, cayenne pepper and parsley.

Cover it and bake at the preheated temperature. Continue on baking until the meat is brown. In about 30 minutes, turn the meat to expose the other side the heat. The whole baking process takes about an hour.

Chicken and Vegetable Salad

Serves 4 with 382 calories per serving

Ingredients:

- 2 cups grilled chicken breast, chopped

- ½ cup carrot, sliced in matchstick julienne

- 1 and ¼ cups cucumber, chopped in the same size as the chicken

- ½ cup radish, sliced in matchstick julienne

- ¼ cup mayonnaise, light

- 1/3 cup green onions, chopped

- 1 teaspoon garlic, minced

- ¼ teaspoon cumin, ground

- Salt and pepper to taste

Instuctions:

Mix the chicken and the vegetables in a large bowl. In a separate bowl, combine the mayonaise and tthe spices. Adjust the taste according to your preference, but limit the salt.

Mix in the mayonnaise mixture to the chicken. Toss the ingredients together until the chicken and the vegetables are coated with the dressing.

Serve with pita bread.

Cucumber and Mango Salad

Serves 4 with 145 calories per serving

Ingredients:

- ½ kilo of cucumber,

- ¾ kilo of ripe mango

- 2 teaspoons of sesame seeds, toasted

- ½ teaspoon of rice vinegar

- 1 teaspoon raw honey or agave nectar

Instructions:

Trim the ends of the cucumber.

Peel half of the cucumber and leave the others unpeeled. (Optional)

Slice the cucumbers into ¼ inch rounds. Arrange in salad bowls.

Cut the mangoes in halves and remove the seed. Scoop out the mangoes and chop it into small bite size pieces. Mix with the cucumber.

In a small bowl, combine the vinegar and honey. Drizzle it over the fruit and vegetable. Toss until everything is coated.

Sprinkle with toasted sesame seeds. Toss lightly and serve.

Chicken Noodle Soup

Serves 5 with 280 calories per serving

Ingredients:

- ¼ pound noodles

- 2 cups shredded chicken breast

- ½ cup celery, chopped

- ¼ cup carrots, diced

- ¼ cup onion, diced

- 2 tablespoon olive oil

- 6 cups chicken stock made from 4 to 5 chicken bouilon and 6 cups water

- ¼ teaspoon of ground pepper and dried marjoram

- 1 ½ teaspoon parsley, chopped

Instructions:

In a deep pot placed over medium heat, sautte the onion using the olive oil until it becomes translucent in color.

Add the celery and continue sauteeing for two minutes. Mix in the chicken and the carrots. Saute for another three minutes.

Pour the chicken stock. Add the marjoram, parsley and a dash of pepper and salt. Bring to a boil . Adjust the taste according to your preference.

Add the noodle and let it simmer for 3 to 5 minutes or according to the package instruction. Serve.

DINNER

Salmon (Tuna) and Fruit salad

Serves 6 with 230 calories per serving

Ingredients:

- Generous amount of salad greens

- 2 300-320 grams canned salmon or albacore tuna (flakes in water)

- 2 ripe large ripe avocados (mashed)

- 1 tsp. sea salt

- 1 tsp. ground pepper

Instructions:

Place the salmon in a serving bowl. Add the mashed avocado and mix. Add pepper then taste. Add pepper and sea salt to taste. Mix thoroughly. Serve together with salad greens.

Baked Tilapia

Serves 6 with 250 calories per serving

Ingredients:

- 900 grams of tilapia fillet

- 4 tbsp. extra virgin olive oil

- 8 tbsp. tamari

- 4 tbsp. unprocessed honey

- 6 garlic cloves

- 1 piece fresh ginger

Instructions:

Mince the garlic. Grate the ginger until you have 3 teaspoons. Mix the ginger, olive oil, honey and garlic in a bowl. Marinate the tilapia fillet in the mixture for one hour in a sealable plastic container. Turn the container once on the 30th minute. Bake the meat in 150 C on a baking pan for 10 minutes. On the 10th minute, flip it and cook for about 5 more minutes.

Baked Chicken and Fruits

Serves 6 with 410 calories per serving

Ingredients:

- 750 grams organic chicken breast

- 1 cup organic mayonnaise or avocado mayonnaise

- 1 cup celery

- 1 medium apple

- 1 small onion

- 5 tsp. curry powder

- 1 tsp. turmeric

- Sea salt to taste

- Pepper to taste

Instructions:

Bake the chicken breasts until cooked and the cut them into cubes. Dice the celery, onion and the apples.

In the serving bowl, add the fruits and vegetables first then the chicken cubes then toss. Add the rest of the ingredients one by one, as you continue to toss. Leave the salt and pepper for last. Add these two when you serve. Before serving, put the tossed salad in the refrigerator for 15 minutes.

This dish is best served with lettuce leaves.

To make the avocado mayonnaise, blend one cup pitted ripe avocado with ½ juice of one lemon, salt and pepper (cayenne is recommended). Gardually add ¼ cup of olive oil until you reach your desired consistency.

Rich Vegetables and Fruit Coleslaw

Serves 3 with 120 calories per serving

Ingredients:

- 2 cups mixture of shredded white and red cabbage

- 2 ½ cups water

- 1 large carrot

- 1 small apple

- ¼ onion

- 1 tbsp. cilantro (As fresh as you can find)

- 1 ½ tbsp. extra-virgin olive oil

- 1 tbsp. red wine vinegar

- ½ tbsp. lemon juice

- ½ tbsp. honey

- ½ tsp. horseradish (from a jar)

- ¼ tsp. onion powder

- ¼ tsp. garlic powder

- Tamari to taste

Instructions:

You should prepare this at least 3 and ½ hours before serving. Chop the onions and shred the apples and carrots. Boil the water. Put the mixed cabbage in a bowl and pour the boiling water over it. Allow the boiling water to cook the cabbage for 4 minutes then drain.

In a mixing bowl, mix all the remaining liquid ingredients. Add the cabbage to the mixture then stir. Add the other solid ingredients as you keep on stirring. Cover the mount of the bowl with plastic cover then store in the fridge for 3 hours. You could let it sit in the cold until it is time to serve.

Cucumber and Onion Salad

Serves 6 with 50 calories per serving

Ingredients:

Salad:

- 4 medium cucumbers
- 1 medium onion

Dressing:

- 2 tbsp. of rice vinegar
- 3 tsp. of olive oil
- Sea salt
- Pepper

Instructions:

Slice the cucumbers and the onion thinly (the onions should be in rings). Put them in a large bowl and mix them evenly. In a small container, mix the vinegar and the olive oil. Add the seasoning ingredients to taste.

Pour the dressing mixture to the mixed cucumber and onion rings. Toss the salad to spread the dressing evenly on the vegetables. Cover the top of the bowl and let it cool in the fridge for 30 minutes to 1 hour before serving.

Tofu soup with Spinach

Serves 6 with 150 calories per serving

Ingredients:

- 8 cups chicken broth

- 3 cups of mushrooms

- 3 leeks, thinly

- 1 tsp. garlic, minced

- 2 tsp. Olive oil

- 250 grams firm tofu

- 1 ½ tbsp. seafood seasoning

- 3 cups fresh spinach leaves

Instructions:

Slice the mushrooms and the leeks. The leeks should be sliced thin. Mince the garlic and slice the tofu into smaller cubes. In a pot, boil the broth and add the sliced garlic, leeks and mushrooms. Let the soup simmer by lowering the heat. Let it simmer for 10-12 minutes.

Roll the tofu in the seafood seasoning. In a skillet, you should heat the olive oil then add the seasoning-covered tofu. Make sure that all the sides of the tofu cubes are seared. When the tofu is thoroughly cooked, add it to the simmering soup. Allow the soup with the tofu to simmer for 4 minutes more. Add the spinach to the broth only when you are ready to serve.

Baked Fillet Mignon with Potatoes

Serve 4 with 510 calories per serve

Ingredients:

- 1 pound of fillet Mignon

- 4 large potatoes, peeled and cut into 1" chunks

- ¼ cup coconut oil

- 1-1/2 cup balsamic vinaigrette

- Onion

- Garlic

- Salt and pepper to taste

Instructions:

Preheat oven to 250 degrees Fahrenheit.

Rub the fillet mignon with garlic, salt and pepper. In an iron skillet over medium heat, add 1 tablespoon of coconut oil. Brown the fillet mignon for two minutes in each side. Set aside to cool.

In the same skillet, add the remaining coconut oil. Saute the onion until translucent. Stir in the potatoes and brown it for about two minutes. Set aside.

Cube the fillet mignon in the same sice as the potatoes. Add the potatoes. Toss until the ingredients are incorporated well. Transfer to a baking dish.

Bake for 45 to 1 hour.

Cauliflower Rice

Serves 1 with 60 calories.

Ingredients:

- 1 cup cauliflower, grated

- 1 teaspoon olive or coconut oil

- 1 small clove of garlic, finely minced

Instructions:

Place a skillet over low heat. Add the coconut oil.

Saute the garlic for until it is cooked. Add the cauliflower rice and saute for three minutes. Serve.

Zucchini Spaghetti with Pesto Sauce

Serves 1 with 75 calories

Ingredients:

- 200 gram zucchini

- 1 teaspoon coconut or olive oil

- Salt and pepper

Instructions:

Cut the zucchini in half. If you have a long zucchini, cut it into 4" in height. Brush each half with oil. Arrange it on a baking sheet. Bake for ten minutes over a preheated 160 degree Celsius oven or until it is firm to touch.

Slice the zucchini in strips or use a mandoline slicer to keep its length.

Heat the left over oil in a skillet. Add the zucchini and toss it for another minute. Serve plain or with pesto sauce.

Note: You can also use pumpkin or squash instead of zucchini. The direction is the same, but the baking period may vary.

Tip: You can also chop the spaghetti into tiny bits and turn it into rice.

Pesto Sauce

Serves 4 with 200 calories per serving

Ingredients:

- ½ cup chopped almonds

- ¾ cups chopped basil

- 1 clove minced garlic

- ¼ cup olive oil

- 1 tablespoon parmesan cheese

- Salt and pepper

Instructions:

Place all the ingredients in the food processor, except for the olive oil and salt and pepper. Blend the ingredients. Gradually add the olive oil as you blend. Stop adding the oil when you reach your desired consistency. Add salt and pepper to taste.

Serve with your zucchini spaghetti.

Grilled Salmon with Cilantro Sauce

Serves for 4 with 530 calories per serving

Ingredients:

- 4 4-oz salmon steaks

- Juice of one half lemon

- 2 cups raw honey or agave nectar

- 2 cloves chopped garlic

- 2 cups cilantro leaves, chopped

- 1 tablespoon of coconut oil

Instructions:

Mix the lemon honey, garlic and cilantro leaves in a saucepan. Place over low heat. Cook until the honey or nectar can be stirred easily and the flavor of garlic and cilantro had infused with the honey. Set aside to cool.

Pat the salmon dry. Arrange in the baking pan or plate. Pour over the honey marinade. Set aside in the fridge for 10 to 15 minutes.

Preheat the outdoor grill on high heat or place a grill skillet over medium heat.

Oil the grill or skillet. Arrange the salmon steak and grill for 5 minutes on each side.

Greek Couscous

Serves 3 with 270 calories per serving

Ingredients:

- ½ cup Israeli couscous or any pearl couscous

- ¼ cup vegetable or chicken broth

- ½ cup water

- ½ cup olives, sliced

- ¼ cup sun-dried tomatoes, chopped

- 1 tablespoon fresh oregano or 1 teaspoon dried oregano

- 1 tablespoon wine vinegar, white wine or rice wine

- 2 tablespoons feta cheese, crumbled

- 2 teaspoons of lemon juice

- 1 cup cooked chick peas

- Dash of salt and pepper

Instructions:

Boil the chicken broth, water and garlic. Stir in the couscous and simmer for 5 minutes until the grain absorbs the water and becomes fluffy. Adjust the heat if necessary. Set aside to cool.

Transfer the cooled couscous in a bowl. Add the chickpeas, olives, tomatoes and feta cheese. Toss until they are mixed.

In a small bowl, mix the vinegar, salt and pepper and lemon juice. Drizzle over the couscous mixture and toss until the grain mixture is coated with the dressing.

Serve.

Grouper Fillet with Tamarind Base Consomme

Serves 4 with 240 serving

- 2 tablespoon of tamarind paste

- 1 liter of water

- 1 large onion, sliced

- 2 cloves garlic

- 1 cup radish, cut into julienne

- Long finger chilis

- Salt and pepper to taste

- 1 bunch of Watercress

- Head of a fish (grouper)

- 4 180 grams grouper fillets

Instruction:

In a deep pot, place the fish head, onion, garlic and tamarind paste. Bring to a boil until the tamarind paste is dissolved.

Add the radish, but reserve ¼ cup for garnish. Stir in the chili.

Simmer for 40 minutes to an hour. Pour the consomme in a strainer and strain the vegetables from the broth.

Meanwhile, rub the fillets with salt and pepper. Heat a teaspoon of olive oil in a wide skillet. Arrange the fillets and grill each side for five minutes

Place a fillet in a deep plate. Arrange some slice radishes on the side.

Take one cup of the consomme. Bring to a boil. Blanch the watercress for a 20 seconds. Strain the consomme and set aside the watercress. Add the consomme back to the rest and strain again to clarify the stock.

Arrange the watercress on top of the fillet. Place some slices of red chilies on top of the watercress (optional).

Pour ¼ of the consomme on the fish.

SNACKS

Low Cholesterol-Low Calorie Blueberry Muffin

Yields 12 muffins with 130 calories each

Ingredients:

- 1 cup blueberries, fresh

- 2 tablespoons melted margarine

- 2 teaspoons baking powder

- 1 and ½ cup of flour, all purpose

- 1 eggwhite

- ½ cup skim milk or non-fat milk

- 1 tablespoon coconut oil

- ½ cup white sugar

- Pinch of salt

Instructions:

Preheat oven to 205 degree Celsius.

Grease a 12-cup muffin pan with the coconut oil.

In a small bowl, place the blueberries. Add ¼ cup of the flour and mix together. Set aside.

In another bowl, beat the egg white and the coconut oil. Add the melted margarine.

In a separate bowl, mix all the dry ingredients and sift. Sift again over the egg white mixture. Mix to moisten the flour. The flour should look lumpy, so do not overmix.

Fold in the blueberries. Separate the blueberries, so that each scoop will have blueberries. Scoop the mixture into the muffin pans. Fill only up to two-thirds of the pan.

Bake for 25 minutes or until the muffin turns golden brown.

Tip: You can also use raspberries and cranberries instead of blueberries. You may also add grated carrots to add more nutrients.

Carrot Sticks with Avocado Dip

Avocado dip serves 6 with 180 calories per serving

Ingredients:

- 1 large avocado, pitted

- 6 ounces shelled edemame

- ½ cup cilantro, tightly packed

- ½ onion

- Juice of one lemon

- 2 tablespoon olive oil

- 1 tablespoon of chili-garlic sauce or chili sauce

- Salt and pepper

Instructions:

Place the edemame, cilantro, onion and chili sauce in a blender or food processor. Pulse it to chop and mix the ingredients. Add the avocado and the lemon juice. Gradually add the olive oil as you blend. Transfer to a jar.

Scoop 2 spoons and serve with carrot sticks.

Boiled Okra and Squash

Serves 1 with 120 calories

Ingredients:

- ½ cup of okra, cut in 1" cubes

- ½ cup of squash, cut in 1" cubes

- 1 clove garlic, minced

- 2/3 cup Vegetable stock or fish stock, plain water may be used as well

- Salt to taste

Instructions:

- Boil the liquid in high heat.

- Add the okra and squash. Bring to a boil. Add the garlic. Lower the heat and simmer for five minutes or until the squash is tender.

- Add salt to taste and serve hot.

Note: This snack can also be served with rice and be a complete lunch meal or breakfast meal. This is a snack that is ideal for athletes that sweats a lot and are prone to joint muscle inflammations. It is also an ideal snack if you ate a light meal, but are high in calories, for breakfast or lunch.

Oven Crisp Sweet Potato

Serves 1 with 90 calories per serving.

Ingredients:

- 1 medium sized sweet potato, raw

- 1 teaspoon sugar

- 1 teaspoon coconut oil

Instructions:

Preheat the oven to 160 degree Celsius.

Using a mandolin slicer or a peeler, slice the sweet potato into thin chips or strips. Wash and pat dry.

Drizzle the coconut oil over the potatoes. Toss until all chips are coated.

Arrange in an oven baking sheet. Bake for 10 minutes. Check the crispiness. If it is not that crispy enough, bake for another 5 or 10 minutes or until the chips attain the crispiness desired.

Take out the crispy sweet potatoes. Sprinkle with sugar and serve.

CONCLUSION

Thank you again for getting this book!

I hope this book was able to help you transition into the anti-inflammation diet.

The next step is to continue your research and design your own anti-inflammation meal plan. Creating and following a meal plan that counters inflammation is the only way for you to deal prevent systemic inflammation. This will prevent common fatal diseases.

Finally, if you enjoyed this book, then I'd like to ask you for a favor, would you be kind enough to leave a review for this book on Amazon? It'd be greatly appreciated!

TEA CLEANSE

7 DAY TEA CLEANSE DIET: HOW TO CHOOSE YOUR DETOX TEAS, BOOST YOUR METABOLISM, LOSE 10 POUNDS A WEEK AND FLUSH OUT TOXINS

INTRODUCTION

This book contains proven steps and strategies on how to choose your own Detox regimen to boost your metabolism, lose ten pounds as well as flush out the toxins in your body.

There are different ways to jumpstart and speed up your weight loss. Have you ever heard of natural fat and calorie burners? No other book can share with you the real secret towards losing the bloat and burning the fat to make sure the weight does not come back.

The artificial way of losing 10 pounds include drinking slimming pills, going to the gym almost every day or starving yourself. Are you tired of trying out any fad diet that comes your way? If you have answered yes, now is payback time. Included in this book are tea cleanse recipes that guarantee the desired weight loss.

This will be a diet program that must be strictly followed to achieve an impressive 10 pound weight loss. Just imagine the different recipes that were designed to be low on the taste part but high in the brand-new you. This program is designed for you to eat food that tastes good while at the same time, does some serious cleansing to your body. It is low in calories yet allows you to feel full.

Be ready to adjust your pants a couple of inches smaller. Several tea recipes and healthy smoothies are provided in this book to make your mornings worth waking up to. They taste so good you will actually forget that you are on a diet. What are you waiting for? Start the 7 Day Tea Cleanse. To weight loss and good skin, this is for you!

CHECK OUT MY OTHER BOOKS

Below you'll find some of my other popular books that are popular on Amazon and Kindle as well.

Tea Cleanse: 7 Day Tea Cleanse Diet: How to Choose Your Detox Teas, Boost Your Metabolism, Lose 10 Pounds a Week and Flush Out Toxins

Whole: 30 Day Whole Food Diet: Whole Foods Cookbook for Beginners, Tasty Recipes to Lose Weight Eating Whole Foods

Diabetes: Step by Step Diabetes Diet to Reverse Diabetes, Lower Your Blood Sugar and Live Well

Bone Broth: Bone Broth Diet Cookbook: Bone Broth Recipes and Guide to Lose Up 15 Pounds, Firm up Your Skin, Reverse Grey Hair and Improve Health in 21 Days

Atkins Diet: Atkins Diet Weight Loss Plan with Delicious Recipes to Permanently Change Yourself

Mediterranean Diet: Recipes and Diet Guide for Weight Loss and Healthy Eating

Ketogenic Diet: Ketogenic Weight Loss Diet, Avoid Mistakes & Live Healthier

Vegan: Vegan Diet Cookbook for Delicious and Healthy Recipes

Made in the USA
Lexington, KY
01 April 2017